How to Cope with Snoring

Easy Ways to Cure and Manage Sleep Apnea

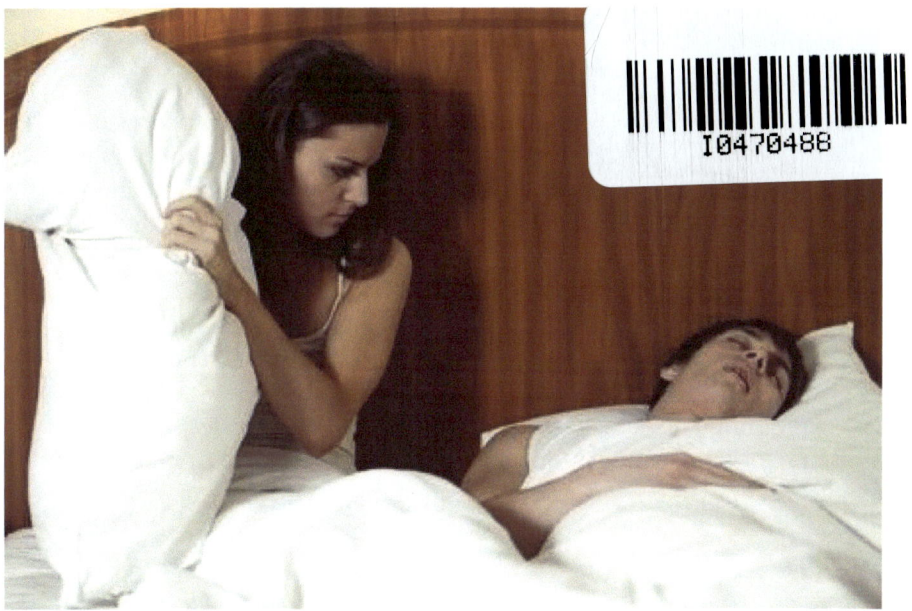

By Dueep J Singh

Health Learning Series
Mendon Cottage Books

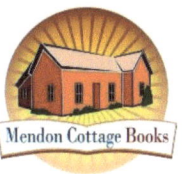

JD-Biz Publishing
Download Free Books!

http://MendonCottageBooks.com

All Rights Reserved.

No part of this publication may be reproduced in any form or by any means, including scanning, photocopying, or otherwise without prior written permission from JD-Biz Corp Copyright © 2015

All Images Licensed by 123RF.com

Disclaimer

The information is this book is provided for informational purposes only. It is not intended to be used and medical advice or a substitute for proper medical treatment by a qualified health care provider. The information is believed to be accurate as presented based on research by the author.

The contents have not been evaluated by the U.S. Food and Drug Administration or any other Government or Health Organization and the contents in this book are not to be used to treat cure or prevent disease.

The author or publisher is not responsible for the use or safety of any diet, procedure or treatment mentioned in this book. The author or publisher is not responsible for errors or omissions that may exist.

Warning

The Book is for informational purposes only and before taking on any diet, treatment or medical procedure it is recommended to consult with your primary care provider.

Our books are available at

1. Amazon.com
2. Barnes and Noble
3. Itunes
4. Kobo
5. Smashwords
6. Google Play Books

Table of Contents

Introduction – Knowing More about Snoring 4

Causes of Snoring 7

How to Prevent Snoring 12

Possible Causes of Sleep Apnea 15

Cures for Sleep Apnea 18

Snoring – When to See A Doctor 26

Effects of Snoring On a Relationship 30

Conclusion 35

Author Bio 37

Publisher 48

Introduction – Knowing More about Snoring

Ask anybody who has had a sleepless night for a couple of days this question – How does he feel? He's going to answer you into a completely irritated manner that he's totally exhausted and he really does not have any time to pay any attention to your fool statements or answer your futile questions. That sort of short tempered and moody unpredictability is one of the most easily recognizable side effects of somebody who has not managed to get his full quota of eight hours of uninterrupted pleasant sleep. And one of the causes of these sleepless nights is the continuous sound of someone in the vicinity or in the room, happily asleep and snoring.

Just imagine that it is 2 o'clock in the morning and you are staring at the ceiling, or at the alarm clock. You have tried stuffing your ears with cotton and even your pillow cannot muffle the sound of snoring reverberating through the room.

Did you know that 30% of the people in their 30s and 40s out there snore? 59% of the people when asked admitted that their partners snored. 59% of the partners immediately replied indignantly that they *did not* snore! But it is true; and snoring is one of the reasons why so many people suffer from sleepless nights and doctors are looking for ways and means in which the snoring sound can be moderated or stopped.

The noise levels have been known to reach up to 38 dB. This decibels comparison can be done, when you compare the sound of a whisper, which is 30 dB and a normal conversation is 60 dB.

Sleep apnea, a condition when you stop breathing while asleep, is one of the side effects of snoring. This book is going to give you tips and techniques on how to manage snoring, prevention of snoring, when is it necessary to see a doctor and if anti-snoring devices are really helpful.

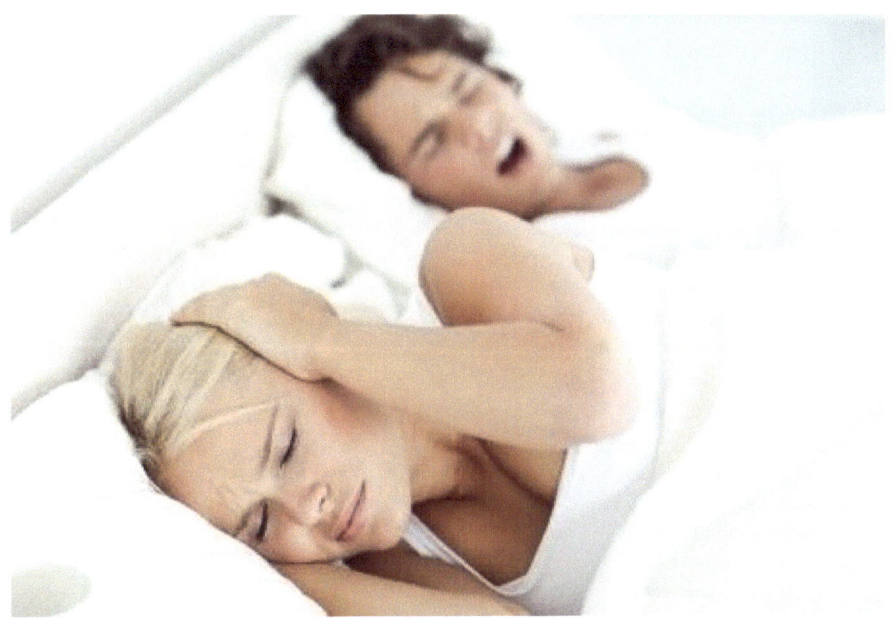

How noisy can you get?

Snoring is a common condition that can affect anyone. 5.6% of children snore, because of obstructed nasal airways. Nevertheless, men are more prone to snoring, and if you are overweight, there is a chance that you are a confirmed snorer and a disturber of sleep for all those people who are trying desperately hard to get to sleep in your bedroom or in your vicinity.

In many cases, snoring is not very serious, and is mostly a nuisance for your partner. Nevertheless, if you are a habitual snorer you not only disrupt the sleep patterns of those close to you, but you also impair your own quality of snooze time. That is because you may wake up suddenly with a snort, thus interrupting your sleep patterns. Many people normally go back to sleep again, and start snoring again, but then this is what happens the moment you drop off into a light or deep sleep.

So if there is anybody in the family, who is causing you sleepless nights, just because he [very rarely she] keeps sawing wood, when you are trying desperately hard to get to sleep, it is time that you looked for the reasons for snoring, and whether it is necessary for a sleep study to be done to see if the snorer is suffering from sleep apnea.

Causes of Snoring

Snoring runs in families. So if you have a family background of obesity as well as snorers, there is a chance that you are also going to be a snorer. Snoring normally occurs when the flow of air through your mouth and nose gets obstructed. This obstruction can be due to tonsillitis, sinus infections, or even if you suffer from allergy. Children with large tonsils and adenoids are going to snore. That is because they have the habit of breathing through their mouths instead of through their nostrils. If you are suffering from a chronic nasal congestion during sleep, you may find yourself snoring.

There is a difference between sleep apnea and snoring. Snoring does not affect the normal quality of your day to day life, when you are awake. That is because you have had a good nights' sleep. It is only that your snoring prevented other people from sleeping. But sleep apnea is when your sleep pattern is interrupted anywhere between 10 to 300 times in one night just imagine waking up 300 times just because you cannot get oxygen in your air passage and you wake up, whooping and gasping for breath.

Snoring once in a while is normal, but if it is frequent, it is going to have a long-term effect on your health as well as on the health of all those suffering from disturbed nights just because you start snoring. The moment you drop off into a light or deep sleep, aid needs to move continuously through your nose and through your mouth. Habitual snorers have bulky tissue growth in their throats or in the nasal passage. This prevents the airflow from moving smoothly through the nose and through the mouth during the exhaling of carbon dioxide and inhaling of oxygen. If the passageway is narrow, the breathing sound comes out as a snorting snore.

People have found out that snorers normally start snoring when they lie down flat on their backs. This obstruction of the nasal passage can immediately cause people to start snoring.

Are you taking drugs and alcohol? Their increased intake can also have an effect on snoring.

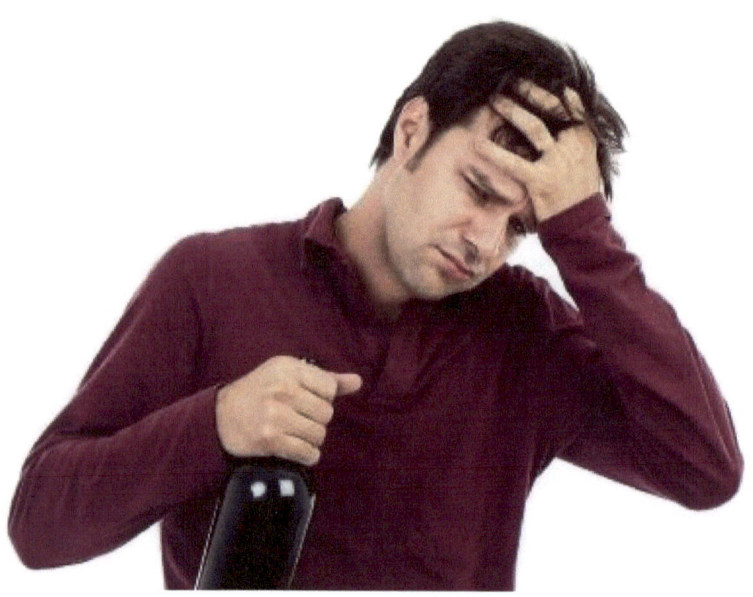

After effects of alcohol apart from present and future ill health and hangovers? Sleep disorders...

I would suggest trying these methods with which you can get to know whether you have a problem with your tongue, with your throat, with your lifestyle, with your diet, with alcohol or whether it is something more serious like sleep apnea. Sleep apnea is a sleeping disorder, which can be potentially life threatening and needs the immediate care of a doctor. But remember that everybody who snores does not suffer from sleep apnea and vice versa. In fact, many people suffering from sleep apnea do not snore at all.

If your snoring is closed mouthed, but still noisy the problem could be with the tongue tissue.

If the snoring is open mouthed, the problem could be due to tonsillitis and the tissues in the throat.

If you start snoring the moment you lie down flat on your back, well, this is a mild case of snoring and it can be cured by a change in lifestyle like no alcohol and no smoking.

If you find yourself snoring in every position, lying on your back, lying on your stomach, lying on your side, it is time to see a doctor. This means that there is the possibility of you suffering from a more severe condition and you need professional treatment in such a case.

How does the poor muscle tone in your throat and tongue cause snoring? If these tongue and throat muscles get too relaxed to age, use of sleeping pills and lots of alcohol consumption, they are going to collapse and fall back into the air way. This is going to block the air passage. This is the reason why you may find yourself snoring after you have had a drink – or two or three – before dinner. And if you are overweight, you are going to be suffering from bulky throat tissue because you have a dew lap and plenty of fat and muscle in that throat region.

Let me explain this. You are fat and you have a proper double chin. You just went to sleep. The fatty tissue, making up your chin relaxed and started pressing on your air passage. That passage got blocked and your lungs are trying their very best to get past that obstruction. Consider the snoring sound to be their way of saying "blockage ahead, signal with sound."

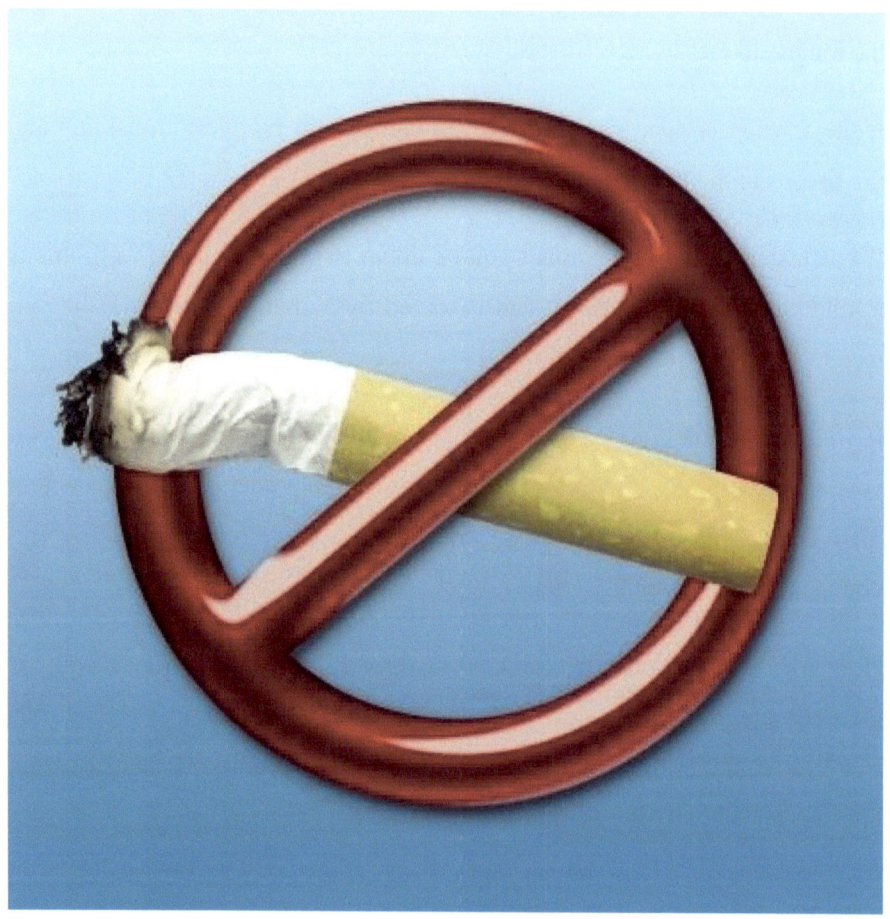

Tobacco alcohol and drug usage cause around 70% of existing body ailments. The rest are genetic or due to other factors.

These are just some of the causes of snoring so a little bit of change in lifestyle can help reduce the noise volume and help keep the peace in the family.

How to Prevent Snoring

Is it possible to prevent snoring? Yes, of course, if the snoring is not due to any factor which cannot be helped, or controlled. But luckily enough, many of the factors which influence snoring can be tackled extremely easily. All you need to have is a little bit of willpower and a little bit of won't power.

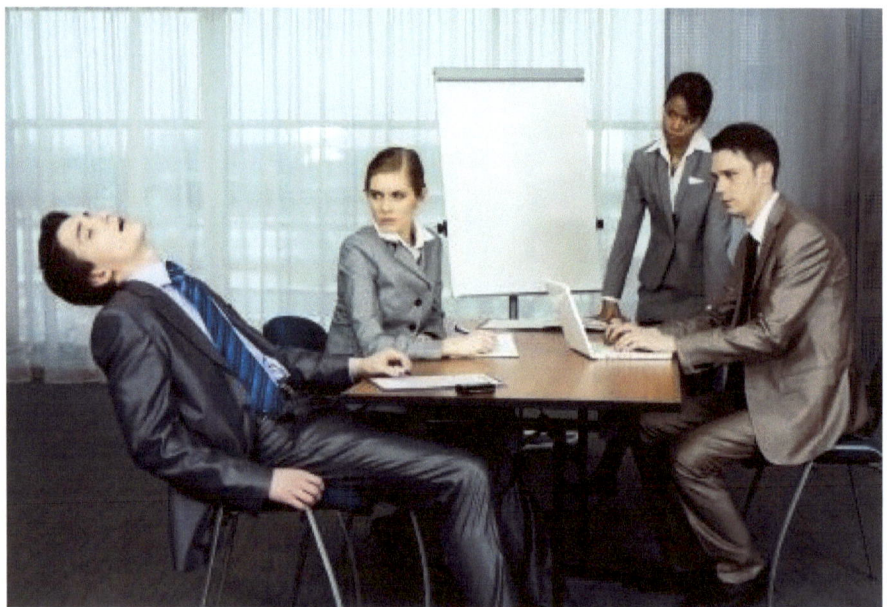

So if you intend to prevent snoring – here are the **I WILLs** that you need to follow –

I Will –

- Stop smoking. (Or at least try to. If I have not started on the coffin nail habit, I get extra pats on the back.)

- Stop the use of alcohol and sedative medicines.

- Manage my weight and try to lose some of the adipose tissue in the chest region as well as in the upper portion of my body.

- I will stop eating midnight snacks and stop drinking that night cap snifter before I go to sleep.

- Take a light meal at dinner time so that my body does not have to digest a heavy meal, and thus stop me from dropping off to sleep as soon as my head hits the bed.

- Try to manage sleeping without a pillow so that my head and neck region does not rest in a position out of alignment with the rest of my body.

- Try to sleep on my side. Sleeping on my back means that I am going to start snoring, the moment I drop off to sleep. That is because my head and my neck are tilted slightly back and that is the reason why the air passage gets blocked. But if I sleep on my side, the neck and the head falls naturally into the best sleep mode position which prevents a proper airflow.

These are just some of these easy to implement tips and techniques which help to prevent snoring.

When you talk about snoring, it is natural that we are going to touch on the subject of sleep apnea and insomnia. These two are sleep disorders, which contribute to a large percentage of people suffering from sleep related problems. Snoring may cause your partner to have sleepless nights.

Insomnia and sleep apnea means that you are going to be suffering from sleepless nights.

So the following chapters are going to tell you about sleep apnea [not to be confused with snoring], its causes, and possible cures for this sleep disorder.

Possible Causes of Sleep Apnea

If there is somebody in the family who suddenly wakes up, because he cannot get the necessary oxygen in his air passages, that is the chance that he is suffering from sleep apnea. Sleep apnea is a disorder, which makes you wake up during the night anywhere between 10 to 300 times, just because you stop breathing for about 10 seconds when you were fast asleep.

A good night's sleep is what everybody and the sleep should be uninterrupted and undisturbed for eight to 10 hours for a normal and healthy human being. However, there are plenty of sleep disorders due to which a person does not sleep so properly. Thanks to this, he feels extremely drowsy throughout the day, and there is a chance that he might even go to sleep, during the day or while driving that is brought up on by sleep deprivation.

- Many people who happen to be overweight may suffer from sleep apnea. It is not very comfortable for a person who is overweight to sleep on his side. And that is the reason why when he's lying upon his back, it is very easy for his air passage to get blocked for about 10 seconds. So it is necessary for you to loose all that excess fat if you happen to be overweight.

- All of us enjoy heavy dinners and plenty of alcohol because it happens to be the holiday season or for any other reason. And because we do not have any intention of walking in the snow, because it is so cold and exercising after a heavy dinner is so passé, , we are going to go to sleep, often inebriated and lying upon our backs, an action conducive to making sure that our air passages gets constricted and we have a completely disturbed sleep. Unfortunately for people who go to sleep in an inebriated condition, they do not know that they are suffering from sleep apnea, and consider the fatigue brought on because of the quality of and quantity of the number of drinks taken and the heaviness and richness of the dinner. That is why drinking alcohol and coffee before you go to sleep is one of the reasons for sleep apnea but you have to recognize this factor.

- Make sure that you sleep, twisted on your side instead of sleeping on your back.
- Don't drink caffeine or alcohol before you go to sleep. Also make sure that you do not use any sedatives, because your duty is to go to sleep without the help of any sleeping tranquilizers.

There happens to be a medical device, which allows you to breathe freely by keeping the air passages open during sleep. It is used during a sleep apnea treatment known as CPAP.

Surgery is only recommended when they are tissues like overgrown muscle, adenoids and tonsils blocking the air passage. That means that there is a constriction in the mouth or the nose, and that doesn't allow oxygen to move about freely in the air passage.

If you stop breathing for about 10 seconds the oxygen in your blood circulation decreases briefly and you need to wake up to get more oxygen. That means you wake up gasping, your heart pounding and feeling sweat up on your forehead. Due to this occurring many times during the night, it is really possible for people who suffer from sleep apnea to suffer from cardiac arrest also because of the pressure upon the heart. The lack of oxygen can also cause a hemorrhage or a stroke. That is why sleep apnea needs to be treated as soon as symptoms are recognized and the major causes pinpointed and medication taken to cure it.

- If you happen to be suffering from a deformity in the bone of the jaw or if there are enlarged tissues present in your mouth, your nose or your throat, they are the reasons why you're going to suffer from sleep apnea. These are cases when you need surgery to remove the cause of obstruction.
- If you happen to drink alcohol, it normally affects the area which controls the breathing mechanism in the brain. So the breathing muscles are relaxed so much that they narrow the air passages and thus cause sleep apnea.
- People who happen to be very fat and have layers of muscle and fat in rolls around their neck, and chin. The moment they lie down, the rolls of fat, press down upon the air passages and the tissues surrounding it. This is quite heavy enough to rock the boat by blocking the air passage. 80% percent of people who suffer from sleep apnea, do not know this reason, so this should be an incentive to make you lose weight.

There are plenty of medicines in the market, which though quite capable of curing you of your disease might have a side effect of affecting your muscles as well as the chemical areas of your brain to make them relax those particular muscles and narrow the passages. That is the reason why many people who take antidepressants, tranquilizers, sedatives, hydrocortisones and other stimulants to cure themselves of anxiety, depression, and insomnia caused by anxiety may find themselves suffering from sleep apnea.

Cures for Sleep Apnea

You happen to be fast asleep and then suddenly you find yourself jerked awake gasping for breath, because you stopped breathing when you were asleep. This disorder is known as sleep apnea and it can be because of a variety of reasons, and a number of factors which are quite like those which influence snoring. However, sleep apnea is a sleep disorder and is distinctively different from snoring. Many habitual snorers do not wake up when they are snoring, unless their own noisy snorts and snores wake them up, but people suffering from sleep apnea cannot sleep uninterruptedly and get eight hours of peaceful, healthy, normal rest.

Sleep apnea can either be mild sleep apnea, when you will not be disturbed more than three or four times a night in your sleep. In drastic and chronic cases, you may suffer from severe sleep apnea, when you keep waking between 200 to 300 times a night, because the moment you fell asleep, your breathing stopped. This can be a potentially life-threatening situation. That is because you are in serious trouble if your lungs do not get oxygen through the inhale – exhale process which has to be completed every three seconds, for a normal healthy person. If that does not happen, you are in serious trouble.

Sleep apnea is normally caused by an obstruction, which suddenly blocks up the oxygen passage, when you are fast asleep lying on your back. That is when the cure prescribed by the doctors to cure sleep apnea, includes changes in your lifestyle, to make sure that you do not feel tension and stress, even when you are asleep when your muscles block up the air passage because they do not know how to relax even when you are asleep. This is done by continuous air pressure upon the airway.

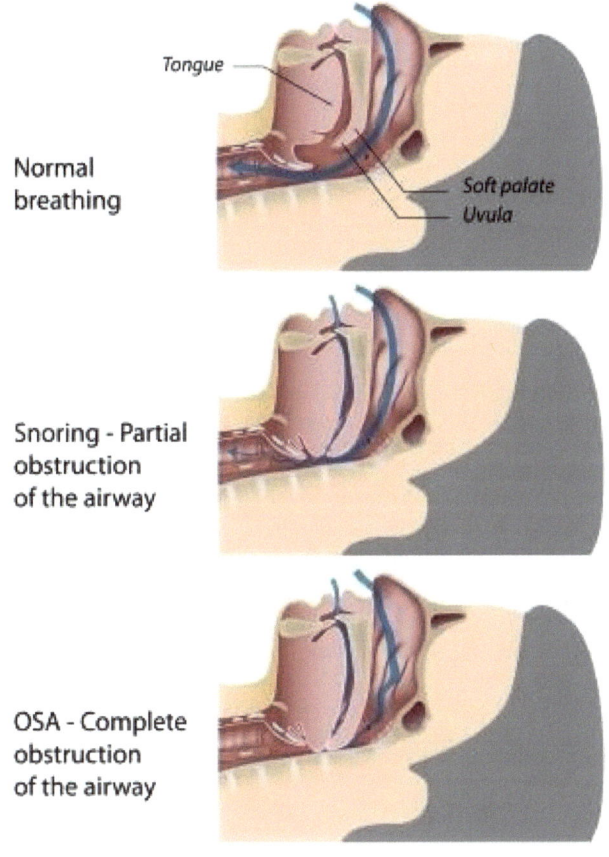

Normal breathing

Snoring - Partial obstruction of the airway

OSA - Complete obstruction of the airway

So… moral of the story- try not to sleep lying on your back …

There are also dental devices which can help you breathe, even when you are asleep, by keeping the air passage open. In the same manner, medicine can also help you, as well as surgery. The treatment is necessary to make sure that your symptoms such as feeling sleepy in the day, because you did not have a good night's rest as well as snoring, and side effects like high blood pressure can be alleviated rather treatment, which is decided by your doctor depending upon the severity of your symptoms of sleep apnea are.

- Surgery only happens to be a last resort when and if your air passage is blocked due to some muscle growth, which can be removed easily surgically. A doctor generally starts with trying to change your lifestyle and uses pressure applications upon your air passage. People who suffer from sinusitis, as well as rhinitis where the nasal passages get inflamed, have to use a spray to make sure that the inflammation is reduced.
- You may have to take some medicine for your thyroid also, if you suffer from hypothyroidism. Sleep apnea can be caused due to adenoids or enlarged tonsils in children, and that is the surgery is normally recommended to get rid of the tonsils.
- To make changes in your lifestyle, you have to follow these practices:
- There is a possibility that excessive weight may cause sleep apnea.
- Research has shown that a loss of weight is proportional to the frequency of your waking up at night, abruptly. That is why it is necessary for you to lose weight, if necessary, to cure your sleep apnea.
- No more late nights; find a regular time to go to sleep and stick to that schedule.
- If you happen to sleep on your side, it is easier for you to breathe, because the lungs force air out, especially when you are sleeping on the right. If you are suffering from sleep apnea in a mild form, make sure that you do not sleep on your back, by stitching the pocket on the back of your sleeping top, and put a hard cover book in it! It is going to make you so uncomfortable when you sleep on your back that you are immediately going to turn onto your side the moment you feel the book

nudging your spinal cord. I found this extremely helpful, especially when I woke myself up snorting myself awake and half remembered echoes of my snores still reverberating in the room.

- If you have a drink of alcohol or coffee before you go to sleep, it is certain that you're going to have a disturbed night. Sedatives and sleeping pills are a definite no-no because they only aggravate your sleep apnea symptoms.
- Viagra happens to be a very popular drug, but it is the worst thing for sleep apnea. If you happen to be a heavy smoker, the tobacco nicotine makes sure that the airway passages collapse through relaxation. This relaxation narrows them. That is the reason why people who smoke and drink alcohol before they go to sleep do not sleep very well.
- If you put bricks to raise your bed head by 15 cm, you're going to sleep at an angle of 80 to 85°, which makes sure that you are not lying straight on your bed, at 90°. Many people put pillows under the bodies and heads to raise the height but that does not work so effectively, as a cervical pillow or bricks under your bed legs.
- If you suffer from mild sleep apnea, it is necessary for you to treat anything which blocks your nasal passage, especially doing a cold, immediately. The rest of these tips also happen to be instrumental in ensuring that you do not suffer from sleep apnea much in the future, if followed regularly.
- Nasal strips are used by people to improve the airflow by widening the nostrils. They might give you a good night's sleep, but they do not treat this as disorder effectively.

What is the difference between insomnia and sleep apnea? If you find it very difficult to get to sleep under any circumstances, you may be suffering from insomnia and if you find yourself jerking awake many times at night, – after you had dropped off to sleep – you may be suffering from sleep apnea. In both cases you need the advice of a doctor right now in order to prevent these sleep disorders from getting to be chronic.

The most common sleep apnea is called obstructive sleep apnea. If the air passage to your nose, throat and mouth gets blocked suddenly, or is narrowed because of some reason, you are going to suffer from sleep apnea.

Remember that enlarged tissue in your neck and throat region was the reason why you snored when you were asleep? This air passage gets blocked suddenly during sleep apnea. This, like in snoring, normally happens when the tongue muscles in the throat muscles relax when you are fast asleep, and blocked the air passages.

You can also suffer from sleep apnea, if you have adenoids or large tonsils. The moment you go to sleep flat on your back, these adenoids or large tonsils are going to press against the back of the airway and block the air passage, by narrowing it. That is the reason why it is necessary to get your tonsils surgically removed so that you do not suffer from sleep apnea.

If you happen to have a jawbone, which is misaligned, probably something like the Hapsburg jaw, which prevents its owners from eating and breathing properly, you're going to suffer from a lack of oxygen. This can cause snoring as well as future sleep apnea. In the same way, if you have some genetic abnormalities in your jaw region, you may find yourself sleeping with an open mouth and snoring through your nose.

You might also suffer from sleep apnea, if you drink a lot of alcohol and eat pretty heavy meals before you go to sleep. The people who suffer from sleep apnea also do not exercise much and are overweight. That is the reason why it is necessary for you to lose weight before you find that the symptoms of sleep apnea are alleviated and reduced.

If you have a very heavy meal and are in an inebriated condition and sleeping on your back, you're not only going to suffer from a hangover on the morrow, but you're going to suffer from waking up at regular intervals, gasping for breath.

Due to sleep apnea, and irregular sleep at night, you find yourself drowsy during the day or often find yourself sleeping at odd hours.

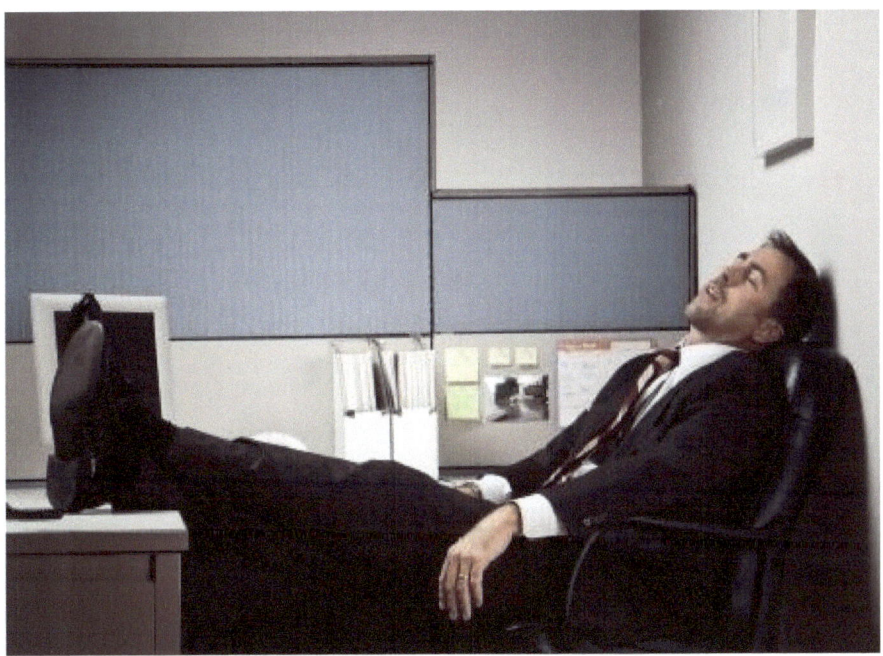

That is the reason why there are so many accidents, because the driver fell asleep at the wheel while driving, because he had not had a good night's rest the previous night. Sleep apnea is also going to make sure that you wake up feeling tired, grumpy, and with a splitting headache, which doesn't quite go away throughout the day and makes you feel even more grumpy and without energy.

It is necessary for you to have a good night's sleep, to make sure that you feel fresh in the morning. If you sleep happens to be interrupted ever so often, you are not going to feel refreshed in the morning. And that is because, you gasp when you are snoring and wake yourself up, you may also stop breathing for 10 seconds or so and then wake up, and your disturbed sleep consists of tossing and turning throughout the night. That is the reason why sleep apnea has to be treated as soon as anyone recognizes these symptoms.

Children who are suffering from sleep apnea, find it pretty difficult to breathe when they are asleep and snore loudly, when they are lying upon their backs, but turning them to their sides make them sleep and more comfortably. Children don't seem to suffer much from sleep deprivation caused due to sleep apnea. However, a child who does not get a good night's sleep does not grow as quickly as the rest of the children his age. He is going to be restless at night, and finds it difficult to go to sleep after he wakes up.

Some of the more current side effects of sleep apnea happened to be –

- chances of heart problems
- High blood pressure
- Depression

- chances of stroke
- Excess fatigue

Doctors usually look at the behavior of the sleep patterns before the diagnosis of sleep apnea is done. He may recommend you to note down your sleep patterns in a sleep study, which is done during one night's rest at the sleep center. Here, your sleeping patterns are noted carefully and the number of times you wake up, as well as the amount of oxygen, which is flowing to your lungs is also noted down. Some doctors may ask you to undergo x-rays and tests also to see if there are any obstructions in any passage as well as any problems, which might be causing sleep apnea.

Snoring – When to See A Doctor

Do you know that a number of people who snore think it below their dignity to go and ask the doctor for the best advice to cure snoring. They are under the impression that this is a sissy sort of problem, and it is going to go away with a change in lifestyle. Well, if you are suffering from a mild case of snoring, it is not necessary for you to go to see a doctor. However, if your family does you that you snore like a factory whistle and continuously throughout the night, do not you think you owe it to them to go and see a doctor? Believe you me, the doctor is not going to smile or smirk when you talk about a cure for snoring. It is possible that he is a snorer himself. So why hesitate, when the cure is there and readily available?

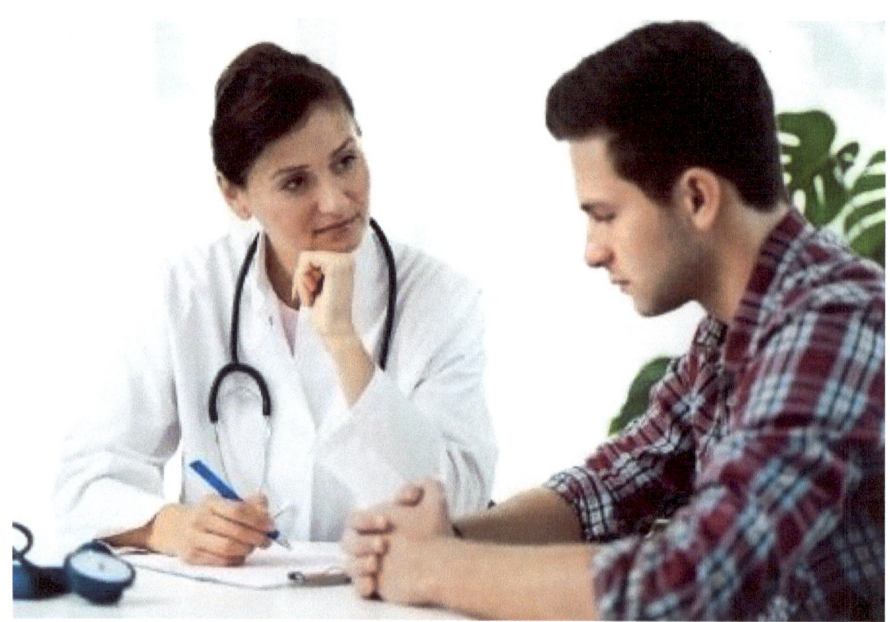

So when do you need to see a doctor?

If you find yourself falling asleep at odd times of the day, – just because you did not have a good night's rest – it could just be possible that you are suffering from sleep apnea or your partner is suffering from snoring.

This loss of sleep may make you feel depressed, irritated, grouchy, and ill tempered. If you cannot sleep at night, you may be suffering from insomnia. See a doctor. The same thing goes for snoring, especially when it is changing your personality from Mr. Happy to Mr. Grouchy.

People suffering from sleep disorders are going to find themselves lacking in concentration and becoming depressed. This is a snowball effect of not being able to sleep properly. You do not rest properly. You feel fatigued. You cannot make proper decisions. You get stressed out. That prevents you from sleeping properly again. That gives rise to sleep disorders like insomnia and sleep apnea. And if snoring is the cause of you suffering from insomnia, get a doctor to give you as well as your part not the best advice, medication and solution.

There are many OTC remedies as well as anti– snoring devices available in the market today and some of them are plainly a laugh riot. In fact, I remember two young enterprising kids making a padded fencing style facemask for their dad through which he could breathe but the sounds were to be muffled and allow them to have a good night's rest. When I asked them what they were making, one of them said "Sound Muffler for dad." And the other one said "Silencer for dad." Now, these kids were talking about a mask, and that is what most doctors are going to recommend to you. So great minds think alike!

Many of the doctors out there are going to give you related medical treatments of which CPAP is the most popular. Here doctors recommend a devise which do not allow your passages to close when you are fast asleep.

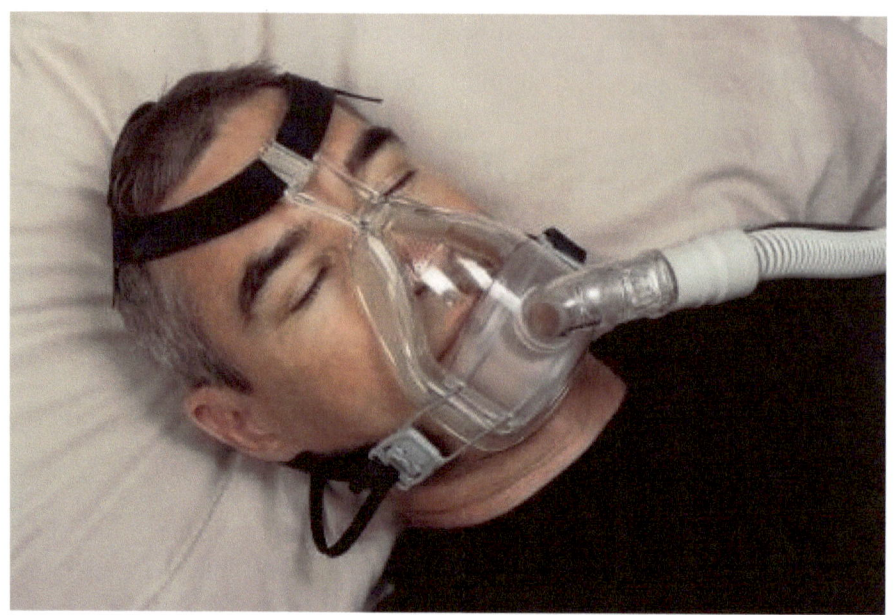

A CPAP Machine helps you to get a good night's sleep.

These breathing devices are normally used to cure severe or moderate cases of snoring and sleep apnea. Some people find it very difficult to adjust to the mask, because they do not want anything covering their faces when they are asleep and subconsciously feel suffocated. Consult your doctor, when you feel like that and he is going to make some more adjustments, or find some other option or mask type to give you relief. Your doctor would like to do a physical examination of your throat and nose and ask questions about your medical history. After he does the sleep study in which he is going to chart out your sleep patterns, he is going to suggest treatment, which may include surgery. This is normally done for people suffering from tonsillitis.

Effects of Snoring On a Relationship

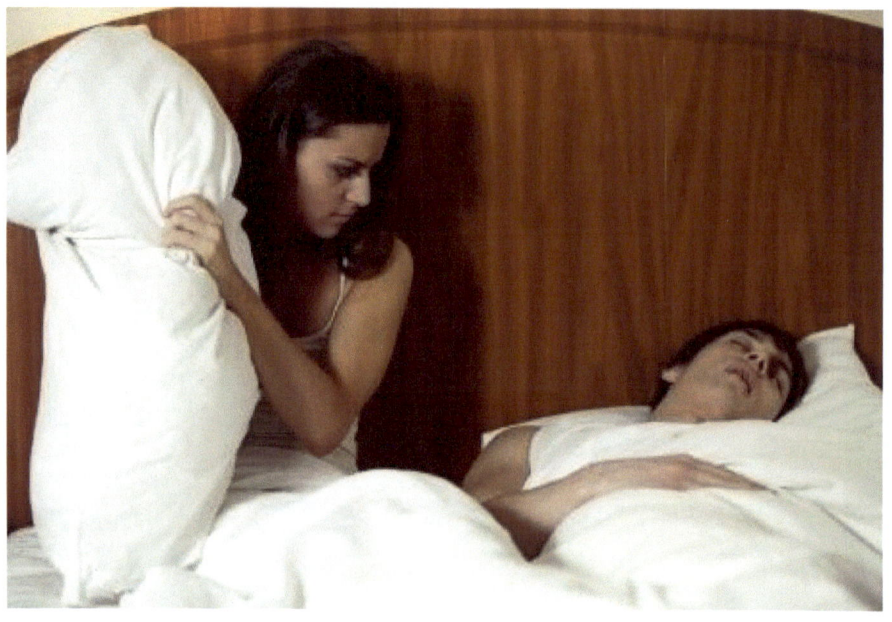

To shut him up with a pillow or not; that is the question...

Did you know that a large percentage of women suing for divorce cited snoring as the reason? Here were they willing to break up their happy family life, just because their partners snored. It may sound trivial, but one needs to look at the psychological effect on why they use this reason for getting a divorce.

Snoring prevents other people from getting a good night's sleep. They find themselves sleep deprived. A couple of weeks of not getting a full night's dose of healthy restorative sleep has an effect on their general health. It also has an effect on their ability to think clearly. That is because their mind is mentally fatigued. Physical fatigue has also left them in a state of perpetual exhaustion. This makes them believe that it is necessary for them to get a divorce and then thankfully they could get a good night's sleep.

Now anybody can ask them – try sleeping in another room. The answer is, the snoring is still so noisy that it disturbs everybody.

Some disgruntled partners may even say that he/she has no interest in curing this problem as long as he gets a good night's sleep. He could not care less about the well-being of his family who cannot sleep. How selfish he is. This is an emotional side effect of not having a good night's rest for a number of days. The idea that you have been put upon, that your partner does not care enough for you, just because he could not look for a solution to cure him of snoring and such other factors come into the mind of anybody suffering from having a partner who snores.

Some women also resort to sleeping pills in order to go to sleep and shut out the sound of snores. This is definitely not an advisable option, because sleeping pills are addictive. Also, the sleep induced by the usage of sleeping pills is not natural sleep. So the option is not divorce, the option is not sleeping pills, but the option is to look at the reason why your partner snores. Would you prefer that he suffered from sleep apnea and woke up gasping for breath, just because his nasal passage is blocked? People with partners suffering from sleep apnea have it worse than people with partners who are snorers. Sleep apnea means disturbed sleep anywhere between 10 – 300 times in a night! Just imagine that. Also, this reminds me of a rather sad story.

I had a relative who had a very loving and successful married relationship with her husband. Throughout the long give-and-take of a happy marriage, we often used to hear her half laughingly complain that the only thing which stopped from being perfect was that he snored. He snored terribly and she had to push him on his side, about 4 to 5 times a night to stop him making all those unmelodious sounds. In answer her husband lovingly used to retort that of course he never snored, but his wife had this bad habit of kicking him and that was from day one, and he indulged her, because she was such a good wife, and she just needed an excuse to get rid of her pent-up anger throughout the day by kicking him at night, and because he was a good husband, he allowed her to do that. And so on and so forth.

Now this was the humor used by mature people who knew how to make their relationship flourish. And we used to look at both of them, and envy that deep love, feeling of absolute trust, sympathy and understanding subconsciously. The husband died a couple of days after they had celebrated their 63rd wedding anniversary. I managed to get to see that lady a couple of months later and I was just talking to her about our lovable Big Papa, who we missed so terribly. And with tears in her eyes, she said," I miss him so much in every way. Most of all, I miss the sound of his loud and companionable snoring. You know sometimes he used to wake up when I used to just nudge him to make him turn over on his side. And his immediate reaction was "I am not snoring, stop kicking me woman." And then he would laugh and go back to sleep and I would look at him sleeping with a smile on his face, and give thanks that he was my husband and we had this togetherness till I dropped off to sleep. Until of course when he started snoring, yet once again." And she started weeping silently.

I was a bit perplexed here. Here was she saying that she missed the snoring, which was companionable? And she used to complain so much about Big Papa's snoring. In fact, it was a loving family joke. We expected her to complain about his snoring on every get-together. We would feel deprived if both of them did not get into an argument about his snoring and the rest of the family enjoying their hilarious and witty give-and-take. She answered, "Seriously speaking, I considered this too small a matter to blow up out of all proportions even though your Big Papa was very noisy when he snored. Many times I used to get very irritated. Once I even recorded the sound of his snoring and switched on the tape recorder, that night the moment he started to snore. And he slept through it. Awful man! But then I loved him for what he was and for what we shared. And I wish he was here so that I could tease him a bit more about his snoring." She finished lovingly and reminiscently.

Now that is what a mature, clear thinking and well-balanced woman believed. She was not going into any temper tantrums just because her sleep was interrupted every day at least 2 to 3 times a night for 63 long years. Imagine that. Instead, she was just glad that she had her man near her and a man who could laugh when his sleep was interrupted by his wife, who nudged him awake. Talk about patience and tolerance of the older generation.

The modern generation does not have that sort of patience and feeling of understanding at all. We could not be glad for someone's loving presence, but we would rather have a commitment broken up because we are not willing to compromise and talk things over. The first instinctive idea is divorce. So before you think of such a drastic step, I would suggest that if you find your relationship deteriorating just because your partner snores, try asking him to see a doctor. Accompany him there, so that he can see that you are giving him your full support. Your doctor is going to give your partner the best treatment and advise on how snoring can be cured in a proper manner.

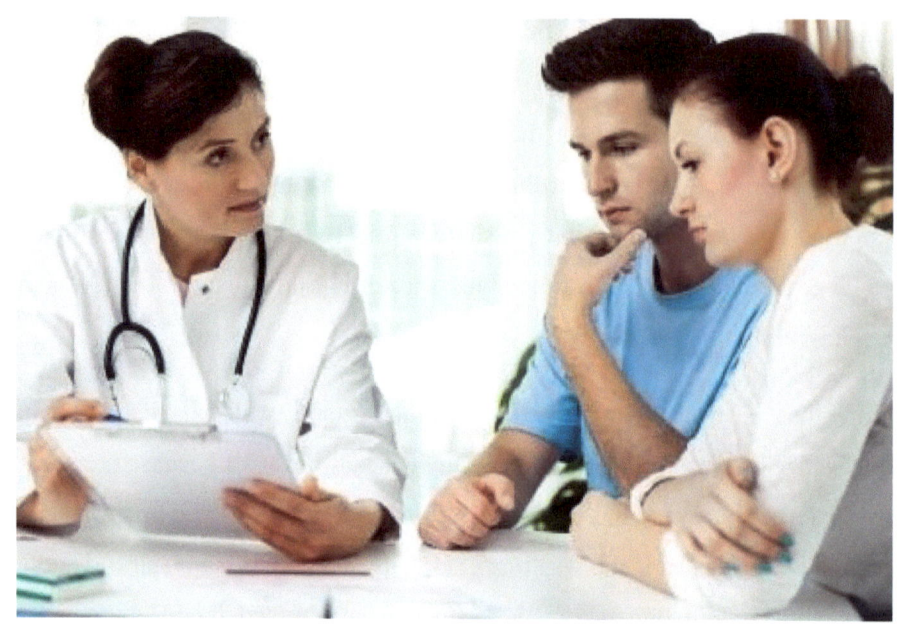

A little bit of familial and professional support keeps families together…

Conclusion

So now that you know all about the reasons for snoring, and you know a little bit about sleep disorders, like insomnia and sleep apnea, you will understand that it is very easy to prevent these problems from changing or taking over your life. A little bit of change in lifestyle, a little bit of help from your friendly neighborhood doctor and you will never have to worry about snoring ever again.

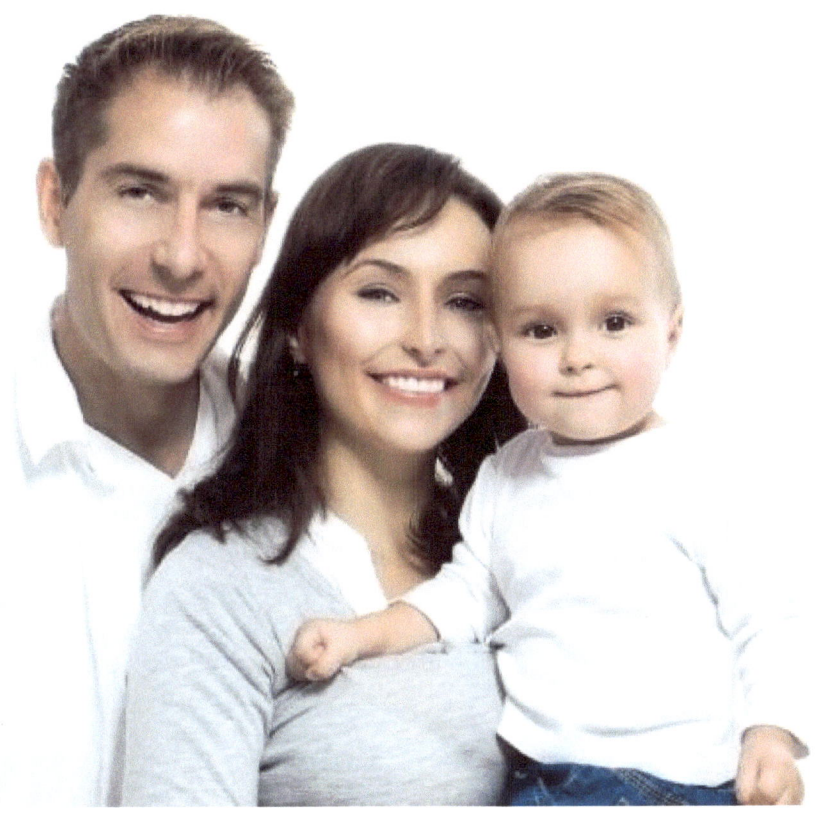

This Is What Life Should Be All about. Good Luck and Best Wishes for a Happy and Healthy Life.

Life is for living Emperor Size. The solutions are out there. So just go out and get the solutions from friends, well-wishers, guides, counselors, and your doctor if necessary. Remember that your health is in your hands so if you neglect it now you are only giving way to future trouble, stress, worry and problems. So if you have somebody in the family who snores or if you are a snorer yourself, or if you are suffering from insomnia or sleep apnea get the right medical treatment or solution right now. It is easy, and so do not let anything come in the way of Good Health, Which Is Your Birthright.

Author Bio

Dueep Jyot Singh is a Management and IT Professional who managed to gather Postgraduate qualifications in Management and English and Degrees in Science, French and Education while pursuing different enjoyable career options like being an hospital administrator, IT,SEO and HRD Database Manager/ trainer, movie scriptwriter, theatre artiste and public speaker, lecturer in French, Marketing and Advertising, ex-Editor of Hearts On Fire (now known as Solctice) Books Missouri USA, advice columnist and cartoonist, publisher and Aviation School trainer, ex- moderator on Medico.in, banker, student councilor ,travelogue writer … among other things! One fine morning, she decided that she had enough of killing herself by Degrees and went back to her first love -- writing. It's more enjoyable! She already has 24 published academic and 11 fiction- in- different- genre books under her belt.

When she is not designing websites or making Graphic design illustrations for clients who want Walt Disney, Norman Rockwell , JJ Grandville or Hed Kandy type illustrations, she is busy browsing in old bookshops for antique books,-she has a mouthwatering collection of priceless First editions and rare books…including R.L. Stevenson, O.Henry, Dornford Yates, Maurice Walsh, C.N.Williamson, and the crown of her collection- Dickens "The Old Curiosity Shop," and so on… Just call her "Renaissance Woman" - collecting herbal remedies, making one of a kind creations in Irish Crochet and Aran knitting, acting like Universal Helping Hand/Agony Aunt, or escaping to her dear mountains for a bit of exploring, collecting herbs and plants , trekking, and rappelling.

Check out some of the other JD-Biz Publishing books

[Gardening Series on Amazon](#)

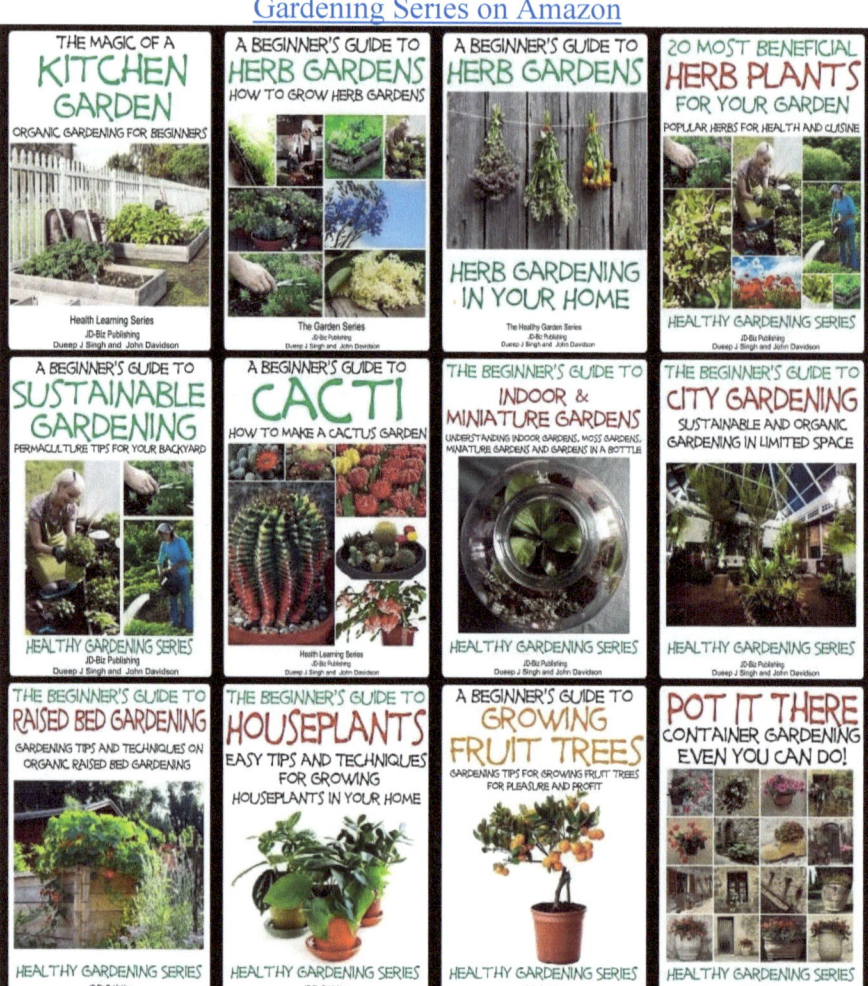

Download Free Books!

http://MendonCottageBooks.com

Health Learning Series

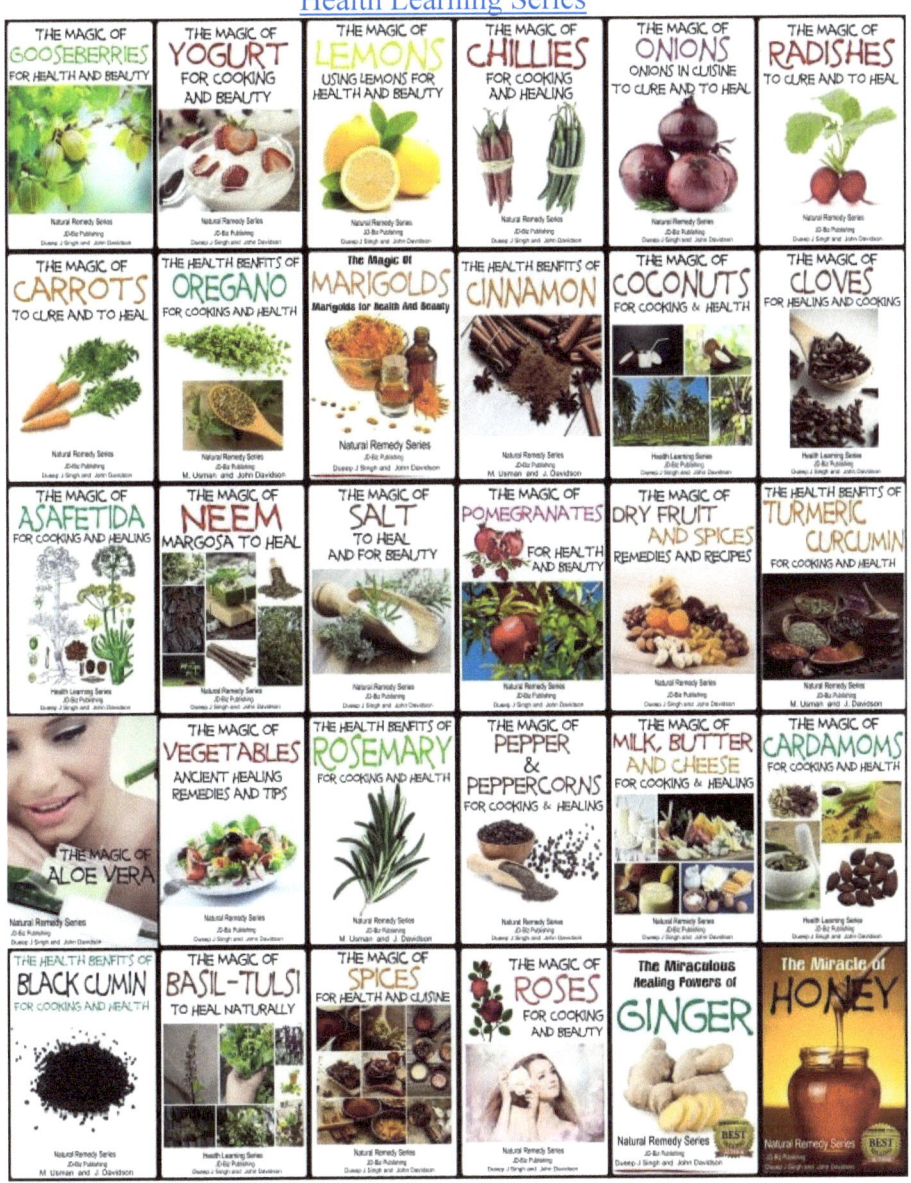

Country Life Books

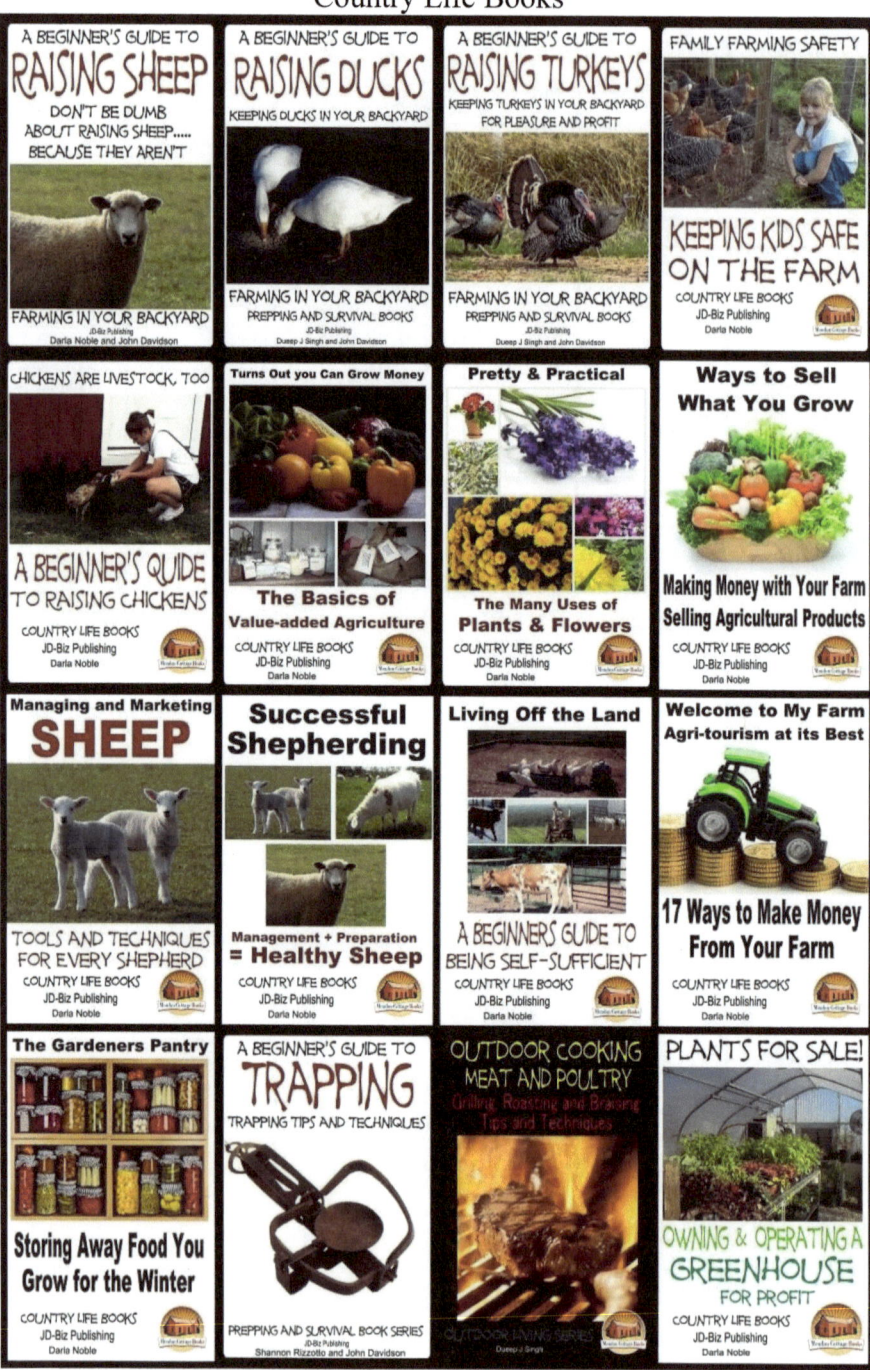

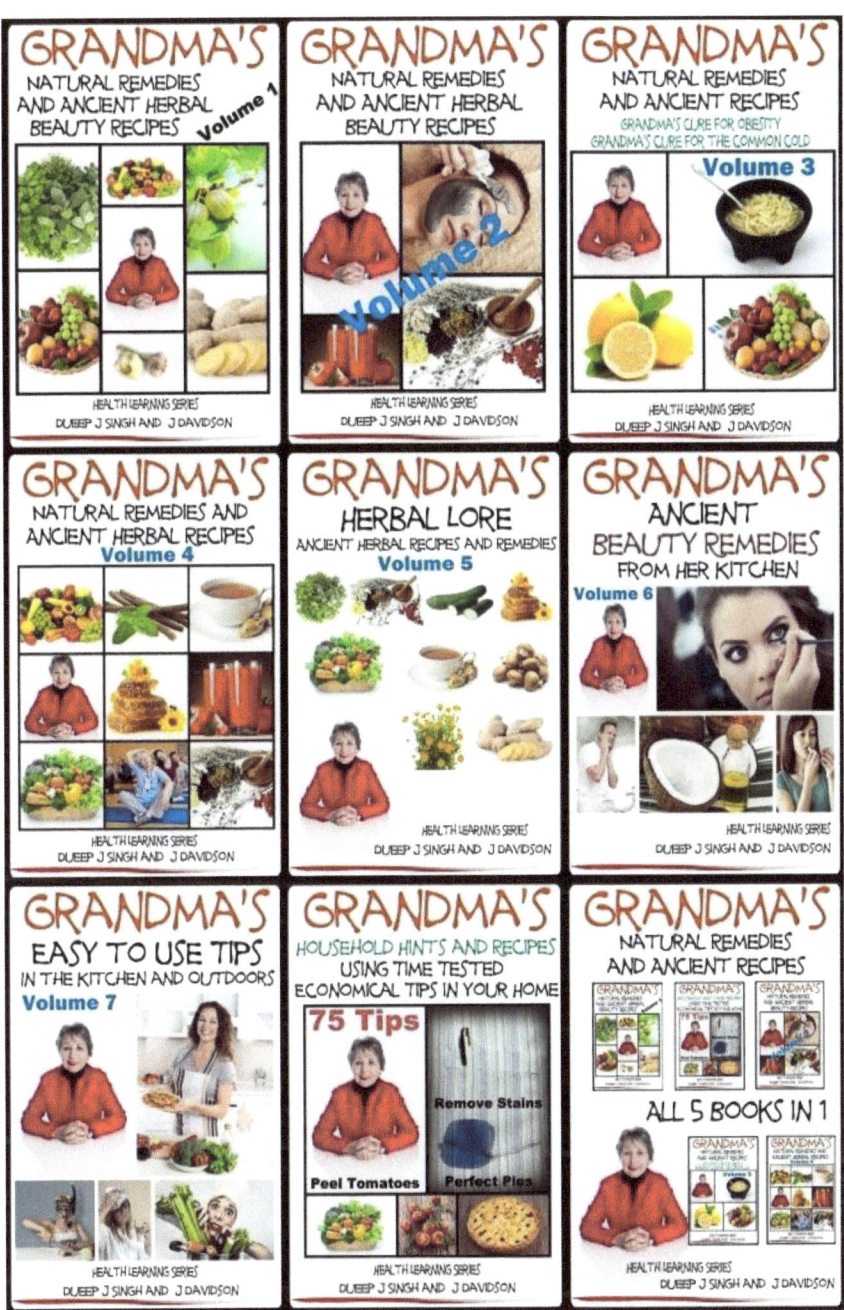

[Health Learning Series](#)

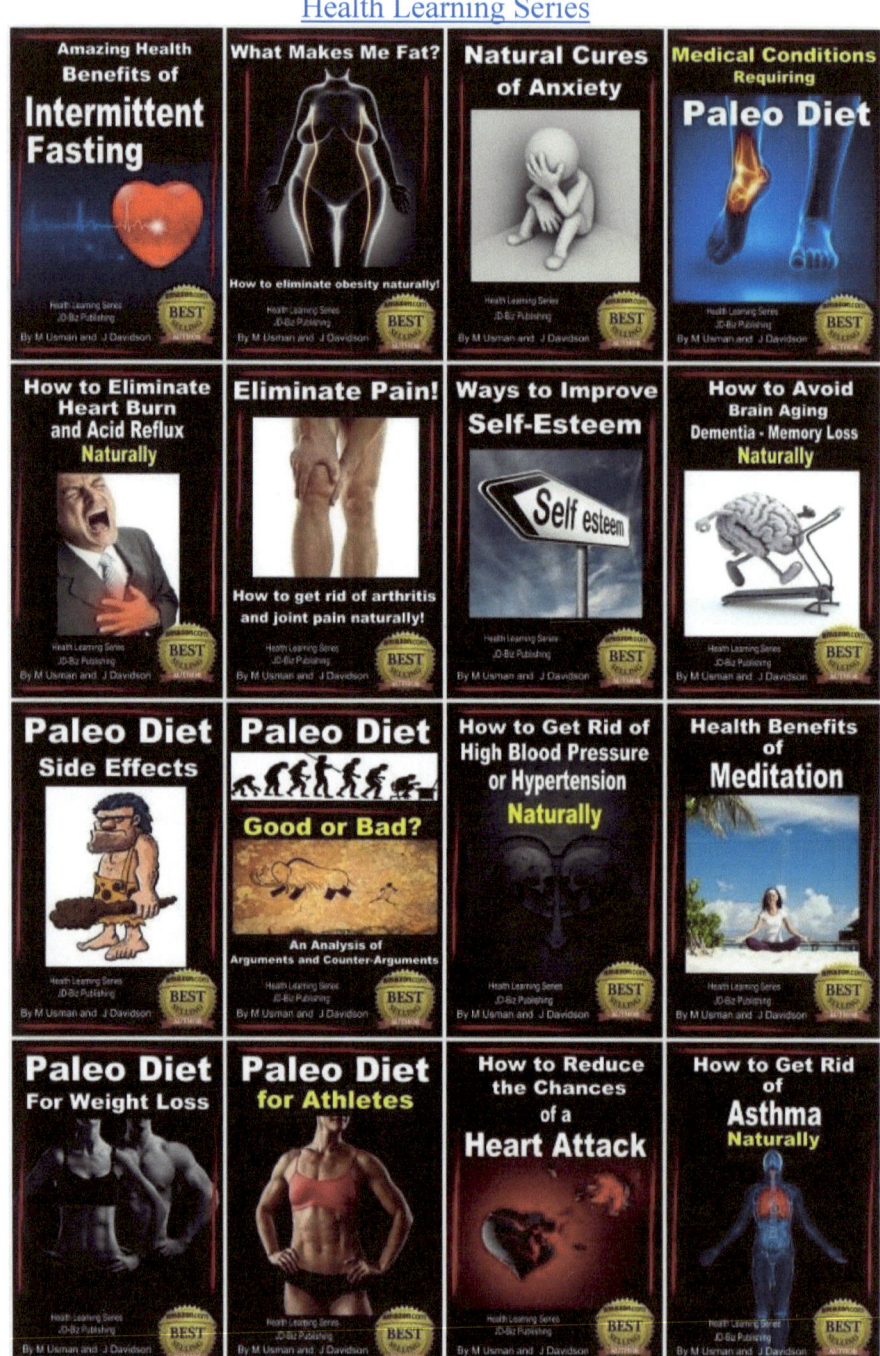

Amazing Animal Book Series

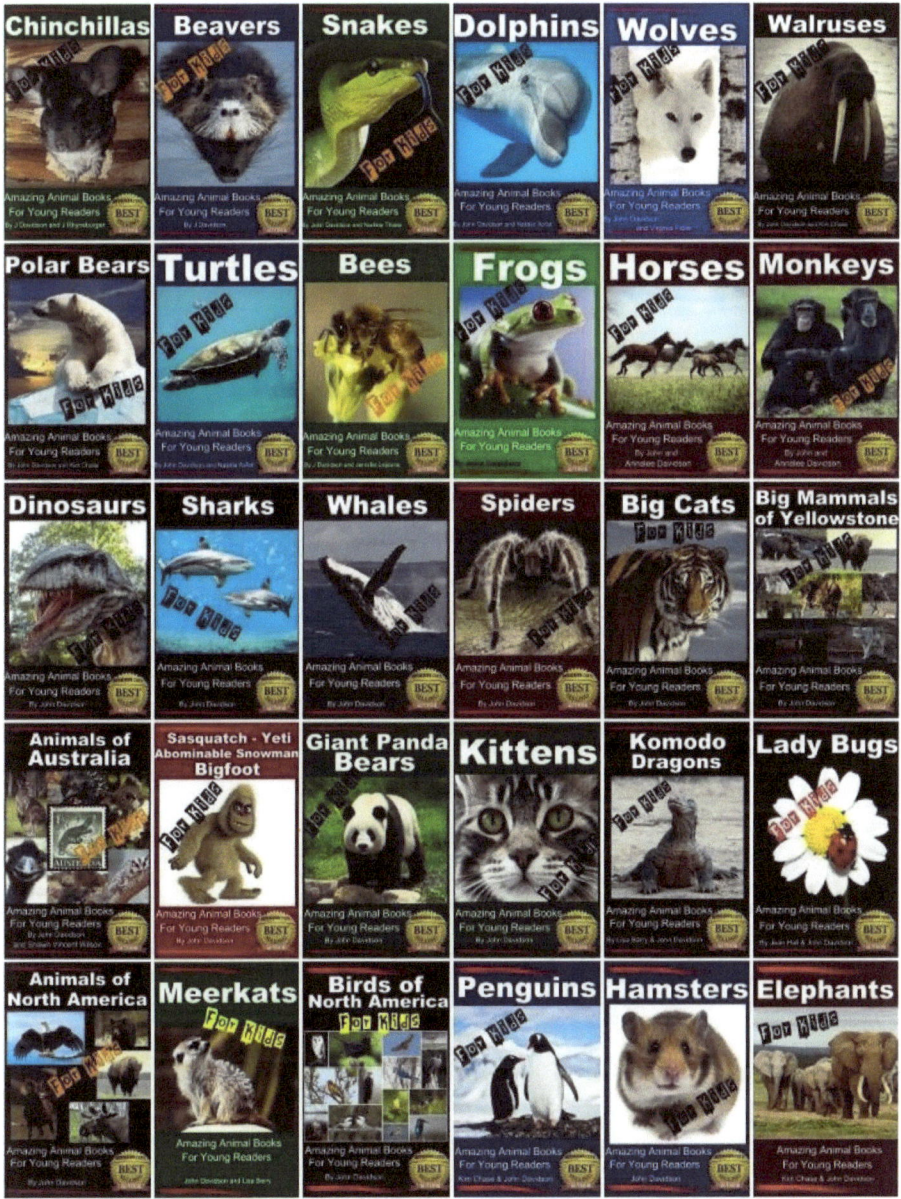

Learn To Draw Series

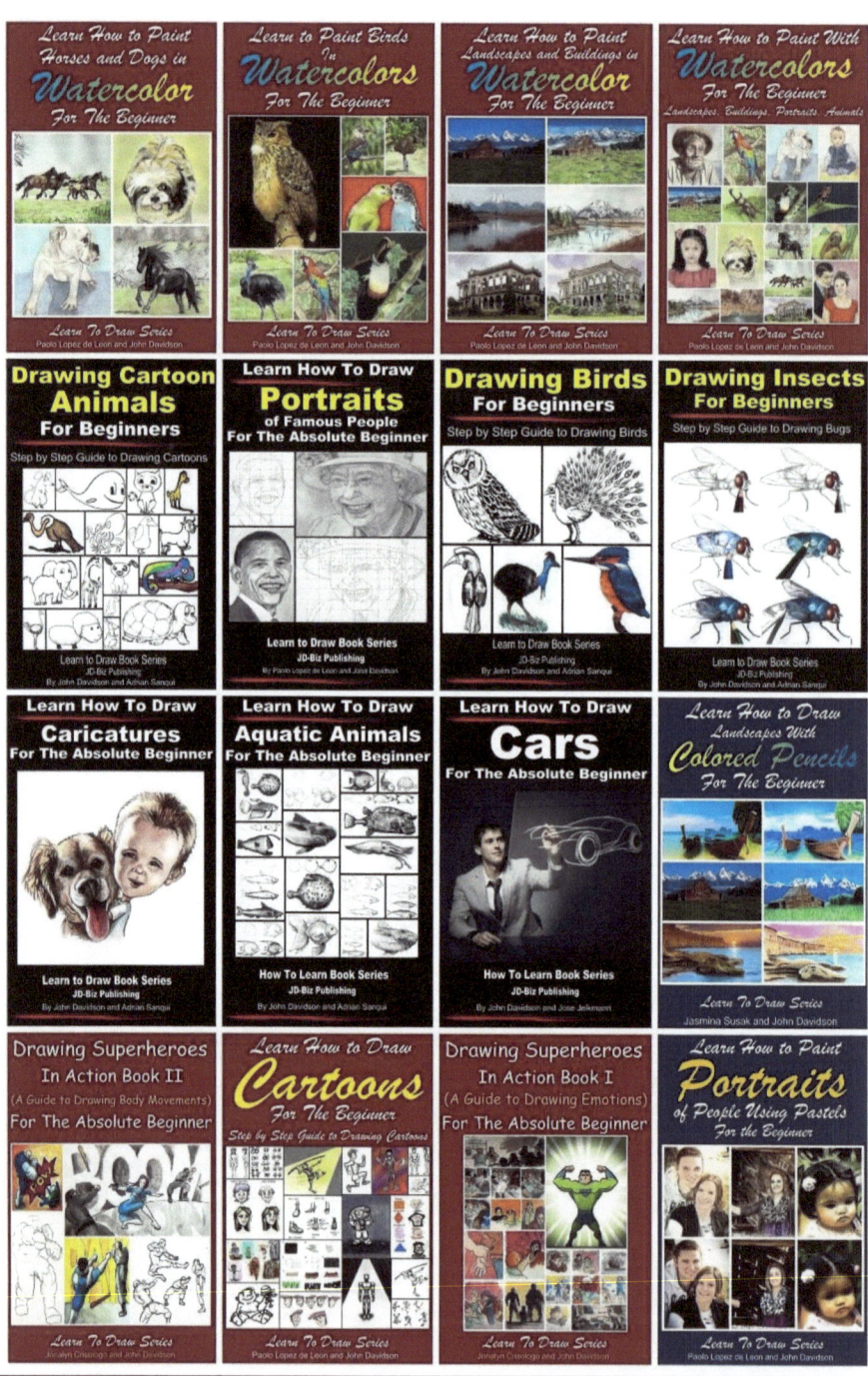

How to Build and Plan Books

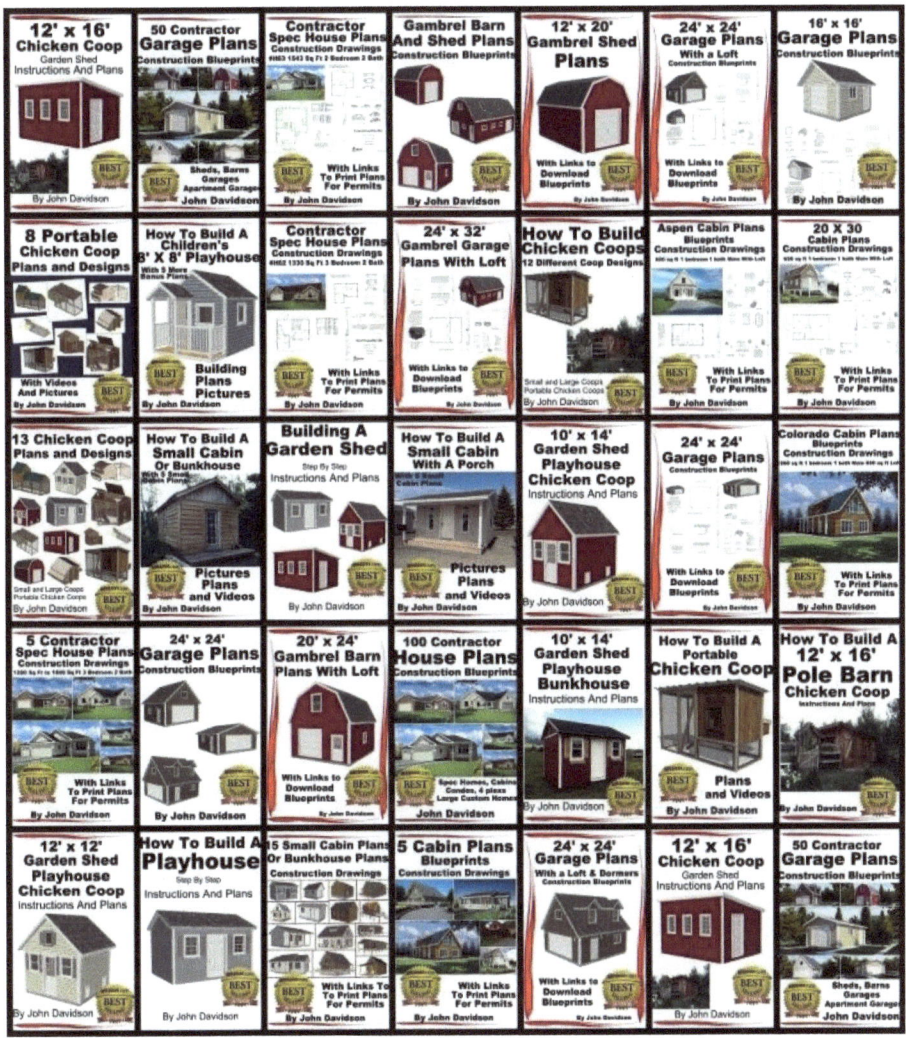

[Entrepreneur Book Series](#)

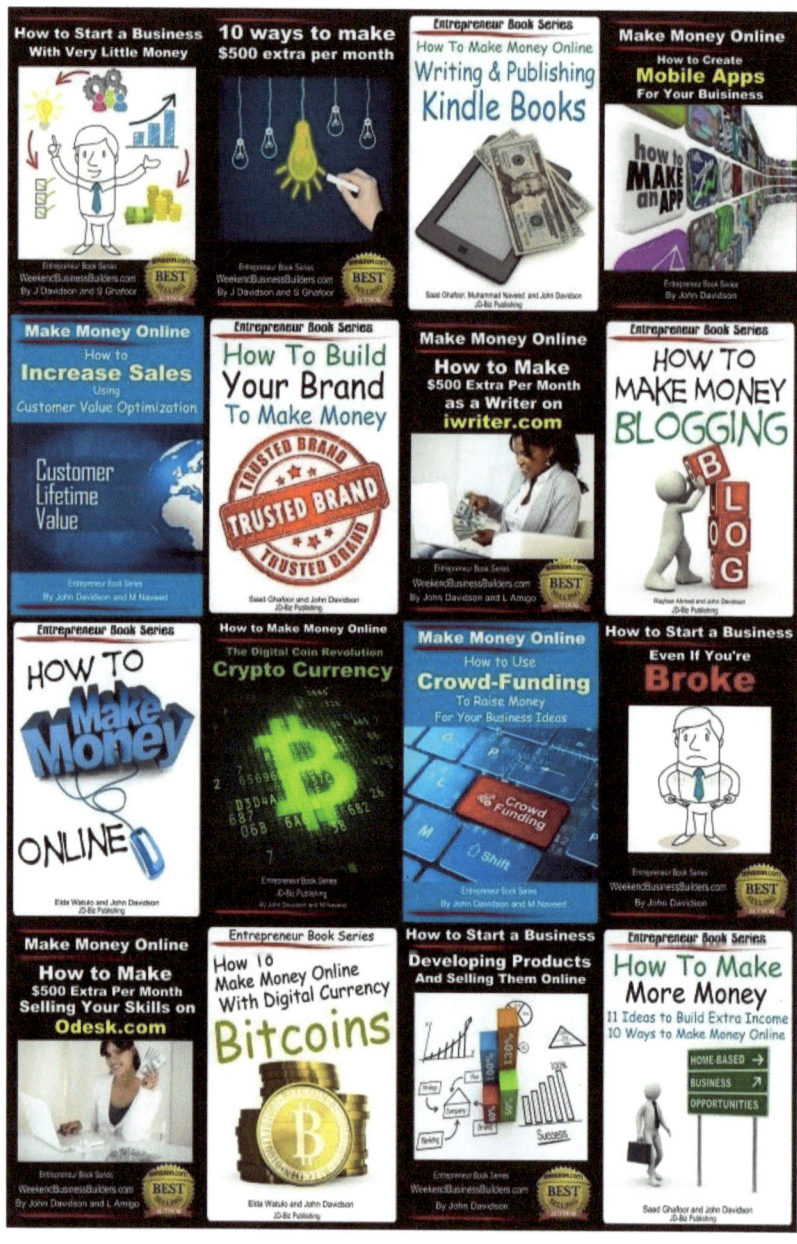

Our books are available at

1. Amazon.com
2. Barnes and Noble
3. Itunes
4. Kobo
5. Smashwords
6. Google Play Books

Download Free Books!

http://MendonCottageBooks.com

Publisher

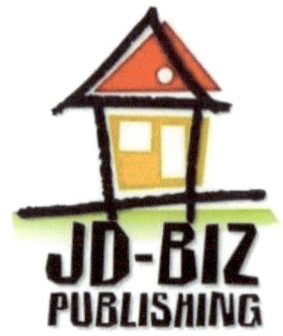

JD-Biz Corp

P O Box 374

Mendon, Utah 84325

http://www.jd-biz.com/

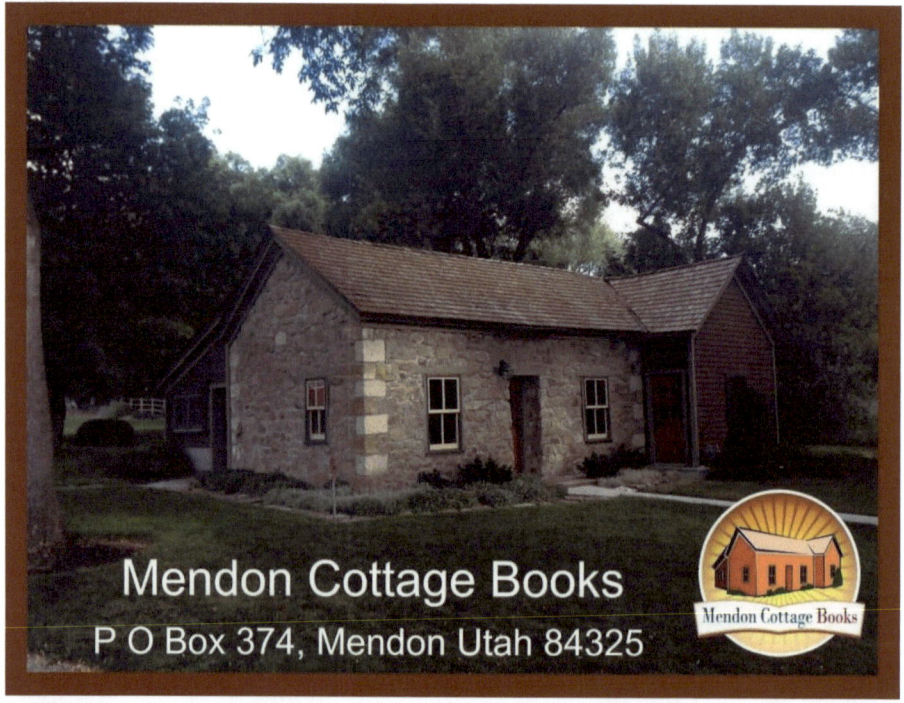

www.ingramcontent.com/pod-product-compliance
Lightning Source LLC
Chambersburg PA
CBHW040922180526
45159CB00002BA/578